Awakening Of the Mindset

Introduction:

 Awakening Of the Mindset Is one of the biggest challenges many people seem to struggle within their inner selves. Learning how to restart your "healing" process isn't easy, as it comes with a lot of challenges and emotions to overcome. To know who you really are and what you are good at, is a start to a healing journey and to change yourself into a new person of what you want to live as. Closing the old doors and finally setting yourself free to do better and be available to the new doors coming toward you. To be in peace and comfort with yourself and not bothered by anyone else.

Chapters:

Chapter 1

Letting Go

It may be old connections, people or situations you are holding on too, and letting go is not easy. It takes a strong person to do so and many of us are strong. Although, many of us deny that we aren't and make that challenge of letting go stronger, rather than moving on. It doesn't matter if it's a person, thing, place or whatever we may be attached too. Know whatever it is, there's always something better. Don't stop yourself from thinking or feeling sorrow. Let these emotions rise and flow to be pure again and find your shine. No matter how long it takes and the number of people to let go. Peace is a better feeling than being around others that only bring trouble. For example, when a child has a broken toy or something they don't like, they rather find something else or get something new. A child doesn't think a toy will become "fixed" or "wait" for it to become better. They will simply find something else. This shows that for many of us, we tend to wait for "someone or something" to get better or fix themselves again. But why be with a person who's damaged and hurt yourself? You have to ask yourself questions that's beneficial and will help you realize what's going on. Think before you do things, think before you say something, think before anything is important and many of us struggle with this step. The first thing you want to do is focus on yourself, health and peace. Yes, people will come into your life once you start focusing on yourself, but it's up to you to keep them in your life or not. Though it is always mostly a test to see if you are determined to pour into yourself, and this is what usually occurs and is ignored by those who want to "focus" on themselves. Getting to know yourself is important and learning to read others like a book, but that is another topic.

Why is it that we tend to be attached to situations, people or things? It can be caused by trauma, mental illness, what a person has to give and more. There are many causes to it, and everybody's story is different. For one to love themselves, they have to go through a challenge that makes them rethink their identity. To realize the real value and truth of reality, relationships, and selfishness. Some have already been through their experience but cannot see the value and potential of knowing their identities.

Also, people who don't know when to leave someone, something alone and don't know when to "stop" simply will not stop. These are the kind of people you want to stay away from, because they are insecure and do not see the value of themselves so they find obsession in anything else. Sometimes, letting go and leaving those who see no value, result in violence. And for that you should never be afraid to defend yourself. It should never come down to violence but if you have to defend yourself do so. Know everyone is not going to be there to save you or protect you. Neither stay by your side and agree with everything, as everyone is not your friend or to trust. Have you ever seen cases where people trusted and were betrayed? Or those who tried to leave someone but were killed or the situation resulted in violence? There are many cases and situations where things have happened all over the world.

So, if you are wanting to let go or leave someone, plan in advance.

Chapter 2

Plan In Advance

To move and understand, you have to plan in advance. Planning in advance is important and has helped many to be successful. Rather it be a career, Job, Party, Hanging with a couple of friends. It could be anything, simple or non-simple, it doesn't matter and no one is too young to plan in advance. Never let anyone's thoughts, minds, and opinions take control of you. Because you should have full control of yourself as well as accountability. For example, the creator of this book is young. A young black girl, rather my color I have learned a lot and been through a lot. So, I take what I learned and benefit from it so I won't make the same mistake again. Which is planning, it can be simple because I "take what I learned so I won't make the same mistake again". I do this because why would I want to make the same mistakes and put myself through something I already experienced? You have to know what to take and what not to take. You hear something? Take it with a grain of salt. It's most likely not true. You want to be successful? Stop stalling and find where to start. You want to be happy and have peace? Stop looking for relationships and adding yourself with those with no value. There is so much you do on a daily basis that you can be planning in advance so you're more scheduled and to become successful. You cannot wait for anyone to help you or give you a push to where and what you want to do or be.

To start and learn with planning in advance, you can start by knowing what you want to eat and do at the start of the day. Yes, plan changes so don't plan too much, let it be simple. You can also get creative with ideas when you have to improvise when needed. Though, sometimes people think too much and be so lost in their thoughts. So, we call them over thinkers, over thinkers are not bad but it can ruin things for others and even sabotage for themselves (further explained in chapter 3). When planning, different ways help different people. Not everyone can plan using only one strategy. So first, is writing down plans during the day to help you be more flexible and prepared. Don't think every day your plans are not going to change. Write what you usually do every day and plans you Want to do that day. And technically, it doesn't have to be written the same day. It could be written the day before or even more days before. That's what planning in advance is all about. Next is Drawing out plans, others may think drawing out their plans is better and helpful because they are visual learners. Like visual learners, they rather have to see the details to know exactly what's the plan and what's going to happen. And last is Reminders, not everything has to be on paper. It's the modern age and we have much better technology.

So, if you have a phone, you can make reminders in your web app or download an app to remind you of things. You do what helps you the most.

Chapter 3

What Is Sabotage?

The original definition of sabotage is deliberately, destroy, damage or poor obstruction. Deliberately is consciously and intentionally; on purpose. Though, not everything is on purpose (deliberately). This usually tends to happen when people overthink all the time. And sometimes when people Overthink, they sabotage what's in front of them. And for this, sometimes things are meant to be sabotaged, people have their different opinions on this but if some things weren't sabotaged. Then certain things couldn't have happened. This also goes into the "Butterfly effect", like sabotage. One thing could change a lot, everything you do changes your perspective and life. It doesn't matter how small it is and what exactly you are doing. Because this is the butterfly effect, similar to sabotage. What's different between the both is that sabotage is meant and butterfly effect is your actions, mind, mental, spiritual and more. It's deeper than Sabotage because it's the universe. How do you use the butterfly effect and sabotage? The butterfly effect is always in use rather consciously or unconsciously. For instance, you are reading this book. This is the butterfly effect, or you may have eaten today, went shopping, met somebody new or even moved things around. That is the butterfly effect, the actions of one's mind and spirit changes so much of life for not only them but also shifts the universe.

And why do people sabotage? There are many reasons as to why one would do such a thing. It could be positive or negative but everyone should have a reason for what they did and why they did it. Sometimes people do it for fun and like to bring others down about it, we call them narcissists. Because they act just like a narcissist, switching things around and ruining things for others and even themselves because they don't like seeing any good and want all the attention on them. The definition of a narcissist is an extreme self-involvement that makes a person ignore the needs of those around them. They always want attention and satisfaction, so sabotaging is usually what they like to do because their goal is for whoever to drop their own needs to focus on them, the narcissist. There are many ways that people can be narcissistic, but we will not go much into that. Watch out for those who seem to enjoy seeing others suffer, because eventually they will like to see you suffer and do everything in their power to make you and others suffer as well. Watch out for those who complain a lot and always have something to say, because they are always looking for attention and problems instead of the goodness seen.

How to deal with those who like sabotaging? There are many ways to deal with those who like to sabotage but it is recommended to leave those who like negativity and spread it around. The reason for this is because they benefit off of nothing.

So, leave those where you met them or cut connections with them. Never think you can change someone for sabotage or in general, never think you can change anyone. No one can change a person unless they decide to change themselves. And this is a problem many people do to think that sabotaging will change someone or make themselves better.

So, stop dealing with those who love sabotaging and acting like a narcissist. Though not all narcissists and sabotaging come from friendship or relationships, they also come from family too. And dealing with family such as your mother, father, uncle and others is more difficult. And there are ways to deal with family members who do these things. But know the more you give attention, the more they feel seen. People who Sabotage and narcissist love attention seeking to the fullest.

Those who sabotage want to be the middle of attention and feel control of situations. The best way to deal with these kinds of people is to not show any sympathy or emotion. This usually makes them feel less powerful and pressured to do more. So yes, they will react more because they want a reaction like an audience to give them attention. But the more you react the more they'll feel good and the worse they will do to feel good and in control of your emotions. Don't let anyone walk over you and use you as a stepping stone to feel better about themselves. Know when to walk away from a situation. Because like everything doesn't need a reaction, know when to pick your battles. Because you will not win every fight with every person. This doesn't mean to just walk away in the middle of a situation. But know the right time to walk away from a situation, because picking your battles and walking away in the middle of an argument will only escalate it further. You have to stay on your toes and keep yourself protected when dealing with dangerous people. And dealing with dangerous people you have to be careful and aware of what's around you. Protect yourself and focus on you more than others.

Chapter 4

Stop Caring

Stop caring, stop letting your days go by loitering your head with everyone's thoughts. Stop caring about individuals and trying to impress those who don't care about you. Stop waiting for texts from a stranger who you are talking to thinking that you and him or her know everything about each other and calling it "love". Because in reality, you are just in love with the notifications and words they are saying. You only care about what that person has to say and so later on you'll end up chasing that stranger instead of pouring into yourself and leveling up. Because once you go off track with caring about others and "strangers" who you think you know really well. It'll all hit you and you'll wonder what you did and what happened, how it happened instead of saying "it is what it is". Because the more you care, the more it will hurt. The less you care, the less it will hurt. And the more you care about a person the more it will hurt because you are setting expectations and getting your own feelings hurt and disappointment in the end. Which in conclusion, secretly makes the other person feel good. Show no reaction, because when you show no reaction that shows others how they have no effect on you. See, people love having control of situations and over people. To be the one and only to control how you feel, love bombing, abuse and more. They want to be in control, and they want to make you feel like you're always in the wrong so you can't speak up for yourself.

So, say what you want, and stop caring who's mad and who's not. Stop caring about "oh but if I say this or that he or she is going to be mad at me and very upset. I'm going to lose friends and they're going to spread rumors about me or everybody is going to hate me". You will be hated regardless, the only person on this planet who cares about you is yourself, you are the only person who will ever love, care and respect yourself. You don't show or teach anyone to respect you, they already know what respect is. They just chose not to respect anyone or anything. If a person doesn't add good energy to your life. Why are they still in your life? There's no such thing as perfection, it doesn't exist. Don't keep someone in your life because you think they have "potential it's an excuse an a ego booster to them for you to just keep holding on. Pour into yourself and level up, if you don't have your driver's license study and attempt to get one. Save up as much money as you can as possible. If you have trouble spending money, put yourself on a budget and put the rest of the money up into a savings account where you should never touch and or hide the rest. But make sure you will always still know where it is. Stop caring and level up for yourself, pour into yourself and yourself only.

People find it hard to do this and to be honest it's understandable. Not everyone has the courage to do this and that means you have to build courage and endurance. Taking little baby steps is good but jumping into everything clueless does not help. And sometimes as adults or children what we've been through most likely molded into who we are now. Though, I believe that can change, because once you master the skills of not caring you will be better in life. Sometimes it takes a hard experience to learn how to stop caring and for one to learn to stay in their place. And everyone is perfect, but because of society everyone does not think so. And because of this society, everyone is not meant to be in everyone's lives. Some are there for a lesson, some have a purpose, some are even there for success and karma to another. But everyone is not going to stay in your life.

So, the moment you stop caring is going to be the moment where you can sit back, relax and realize much more than if you would've cared. Because you will start to realize that people always have an "excuse" for the wrong doings that they choose to do.

Being Nonchalant and not caring are similar but different. Nonchalant is appearing or feeling calm and relaxed; not displaying interest, enthusiasm, or anxiety. Not caring is being un-bothered by things and events that aren't serious. A lot of people want to be "Nonchalant" or "claim" they're nonchalant and try to act as if they don't care. Though it's forced, which makes them or you seem as if you care the most. If you don't care about someone or something to the slightest, stop mentioning it. Constantly speaking about something or someone will make you seem like you care about it more and eventually you'll think about it constantly to the point where it will actually start to bother you. If you need to write down a problem that made you feel some type of way then do it. Express how you feel to yourself and your true feelings. That doesn't mean you still can't express to whoever hurt you or made you feel uncomfortable but remember. They know exactly what they did and they thought about it before doing it, they just didn't care enough to stop. So don't waste your breath on someone who already showed you they don't care once with their actions. No one wants to look like a fool. It doesn't matter what people see because they only see the outside and. So never think everything is sweet and they're living the most beautiful best life because of what you see. The outside is always different from the inside.

Chapter 5

Focus

Focus, if you want to know yourself more and become successful. Focus, a lot of celebrities focus on what they want to do and achieve instead of focusing on others and interacting that's not going to get them where they need to be at. Don't you like money, or love money? Everyone wants to make money, because you need it. In order to keep up with what you have, you need to make money. And that's what a lot of people, celebrities, and businesses continue to do. You can never have too much money. And if you are determined to focus on yourself, you get money before pleasure. Meaning you do what's making you money and get uncomfortable to fill your pockets up. You have to be ready to sacrifice a lot of things to get where you need to be. Sleep, food, items, feet hurting and more because reality is all about survival. You need to have everything you worked for, before switching to something pleasant. You do what brings you joy and allows you to rest, though it should still be making you money. For example, you can make money at any age. And if you really want to be successful you should be making money now if you are young. By the time you get older, you'll have everything you need. Stop spending so much money on name brand clothing and products, don't waste money on things that are not beneficial. The creator of this book, I've had that problem. Spending what I had on name brand items, and products that weren't beneficial. Until I spent it all and realized I was more focused on my "wants" than my "needs". And naturally, a lot of people are more driven to their "wants" instead of "needs". And that's a habit that has to be broken. The more you spend on wants you will never spend on needs. And the more you spend on non-beneficial items and instead of what you need the less you will be successful, because you have to think like a cheap rich person. Have you ever noticed how the richest people are always cheap and barely ever own anything named brand? Only when they treat themselves and that's still very rare. They focus on buying land, building a company, houses and what leads them to money. And for that you have to build a mindset like a cheap rich person.

To be Focus and Successful it starts with changing the mindset. You can change physically on the outside all you want but if your mindset has not changed you will always be the same person. That's what a lot of people struggle and fail to start at. Without changing your attitude and the people who you hang around you will always be the same old you. Because who you hang with and how you act changes your mindset and shows who you are. Want an example? If a bunch of dumb people hang around one intelligent person, eventually that intelligent person will lose what they know and will eventually become dumb like the others. Or if a bunch of broke men hang around a nice-looking rich man, eventually that nice looking rich man will become broke like the other men he hangs around with. The point of Focus is to be different and stop being like the others. Stop caring about what others have to think and say. Opinions can't change and control you unless you let it happen. And even if you have to lose a few people and those you care about, lose them. Peace and self-respect come first, you can't say you "respect yourself" when you are letting others disrespect you and bring you down with them. Not only this but stop telling others what's going on in your life and what you have upcoming next. Everybody is not joyful and like seeing others win. Stop posting everything on social media and stop being the center of attention. Move in silence and be secretive, don't worry about others guessing what you are up to. It's your business to keep it like that, even if you have a loved one or a partner who you are in a relationship with. They shouldn't know too much about you, it doesn't matter how long you two have been together. Think about it, there are things you don't know about your partner that you think you do. Because simply you will never know, you can think all you want but don't think everyone is loyal and is going to tell you the truth. Because you should be one step ahead of everyone, actually be even two steps ahead of everyone. Nothing should phase you because you already know.

Staying Focused means always staying on top of yourself to achieve your goals. This doesn't mean to hop into relationships and friendships while trying to work on one thing. Be ready to sacrifice relationships and friendships between people too. Nobody is always going to agree with you, your actions and mindset. Even family members may not agree, and that's when you should push even further to achieve your goals and your goals only. You have to be prepared for the battle and challenges to obtain your best self. And motivation isn't always going to keep you motivated, so don't rely on motivation to push through many challenges. You have to keep working and force yourself to continue, but know it is important to take a rest too. If you need a rest, take it. Individuals think if you are focusing on a goal or yourself you can't take a rest. But if you don't take a rest eventually, you'll end up stopping your progress and revert to what you were doing before becoming too tired and not letting your mind rest for a bit. Don't overwork yourself but overcome yourself instead. Prove to yourself that you can develop new skills and learn new things. See what skills need practice and work on it. While learning and finding new interests to dig in. Do research and study more to become more intelligent, and watch more learning shows to help you gather greater knowledge. Switch the music you listen to and discover new artists and music to calm the mind and feel more relaxed. Because music has a big influence on who we are and especially our mindset. And lastingly, if you can take the time to be alone take it. It could be taking a walk outside, alone in your room, bathroom, basement, closet. Wherever you feel most comfortable at being alone, take advantage to relax and gather back your mind to stay awake and focus. Have peace within yourself.

Chapter 6

Know your skills

Know what you are good at and what you are not good at. You have to pick your battles carefully and play them right. You should know yourself more than anyone else. And if you don't know yourself and you don't know what you are good at. Get out of your comfort zone and try activities to get the understanding of what you can do. Learn your skills and learn the power of knowledge. The more you learn, the more you will know. Take life carefully and as lessons because throughout your journey of living you will learn and experience a lot which will help you in growth. Knowing your skills doesn't have to be extreme, it can be cooking, learning a school subject, mechanical, learning how to make your own products and more. You just have to set your mind to what you want to learn and not be stuck on one thing. Expand your knowledge and what you want to know, because what if you need to learn something for the future? You have to think ahead and be ahead of those around you. Learning takes time and patience so while you're getting to know what you're good at, be patient && learn slowly. And once you learn, stick to what you know before expanding to other skills.

When you start to know and develop skills. You'll feel better about yourself and want to expand them more. Though If you are beginning to expand your learning. Take it slow and rearrange those skills as "Goals". To set your mind upon one and to get started. You can also create an idea and a reason to "why" and "what it is" that you are going to learn. With this you can start to make changes and measurable improvements throughout your learning to liking. And each time you change your skills into "Goals" and create a "why". You'll eventually get better and better at what you are aiming for with increasing your knowledge.

So, stick to what you know rather than aim for something you want to know. It's like saying "expect the unexpected" because you will expect the unexpected when developing new skills. And learning new skills isn't just for fun, some skills are learned for sports or to just share with others. Develop skills that will last you a lifetime. It can be survival, managing, medical, anything of your choice. But when you think, think logically and act on what's worth it.

Survival:

Surviving is one important skill we should have knowledge on. Anything could happen at any given time. It is important to make sure we are prepared and have the knowledge of what to do in the right situations. Not everyone has good survival skills and knows what to do when necessary. Some are taught at a young age and others may have access to resources like social media and YouTube to educate. It doesn't matter what kind of resources are available. Everyone should be educated to know how to survive in certain situations and have enough knowledge to last them a lifetime.

Managing:

Not everyone has good management skills in managing. It takes a lot of practice and discipline to be good at managing something. In order to have certain careers, you have to know the importance of management the right way and how to use them. Budgeting is also a part of managing and many should consider learning both before deciding on a decision to stabilize in a general lifestyle. It's all knowing how to do something and doing it the right way. There are many classes a person can take and learn from to get the hang of something so difficult. Although classes can cost a lot of money, they are beneficial but can also cause problems with managing money. Therefore, you have self-taught ways to learn how to give yourself a budget and manage what you want to do. For example, if working or receiving money, save about 50% to 70% of money. This is so the other half of the money you have, you can spend on products you need or treat yourself to something. Another example for budgeting is stacking envelopes, this is giving yourself a monthly budget on spending products. The goal of this method is to save more of what you spend. The budget has to be reasonable and realistic, and the money saved in the envelopes have to be more of what you spend. This should not be touched until the end of the year or month.

Medical

Working or being in medical care is a major part of life. Most people go to classes to learn and know what to do in emergency situations. Without the knowledge of medicine and medical procedures. Hospitals and medical professionals cannot and would not hire a person who does not know what to do in situations that need such care. This career requires a lot of discipline, dedication, commitment and degrees to finish and continue.

Cooking

Everyone loves cooking and eating good meals. But not everyone is good at it and knows how to cook. As a chef who is confident in their skills, is able to go out and cook for others, this is because they practiced and learned what will make them better. Cooking takes practice and learning, though everyone has to start somewhere. So even if one's cooking is not the best, it's progress to getting better instead. Cooking classes and school clubs that take cooking is always an option and an opportunity for those who want to become better. A cooking skill is a great skill to not rely on anyone else and to be able to create your own meals.

Any of your choice

Now there are many jobs that require skills and the way we live also requires skills.

So, there's no excuse for anything you want to do because you're unskilled. Every individual has a skill that they are capable of attaining. Now these examples were to explain the concept of being skilled in different ways. Not everything is going to be meant for one person so it's important that you find your own. When you manage to find your skills, expand and improve creatively to become better than who you are.

Chapter 7

Moving Forward

Get out of the pass and move on from those who you let go of. Break loose from the chains that's been holding you back from making big decisions. Grow up and realize, moving forward is better than moving backwards. The pass is the pass and you cannot change that, nor can you change the future. The only timeline that matters with your actions is the present. So do better in the present and stop worrying about the future and the past. What's done is done and there's no going back. The moment you wonder how things "could've " been better is the moment you realize things couldn't have been better staying in one damaged place. Get rid of old memories that hurt you and keep you from healing. Delete and remove old people from your life, and never let them back in. You do not have to say anything to anyone who you are removing from your life. Because once you open your mouth about "leaving" and "moving on ". They will do everything in their power to keep you from success. Move in silence. Not everyone is meant to know what's going on in your life. It doesn't matter who they are, keep people out of your business. Move forward and live the dream you want to live as. Don't think about the dream, be the dream.

Moving forward is all about getting closer to God (If you are religious) or being better and more educated. It's like a new makeover of your personality and self-respect. As spoken in chapter 5 "Focus", you are becoming New. Leaving the old person and the life you used to live in the past. And opening new doors to a life that will be luxurious. There will be no more chasing and changing who you want to be. Once you learn to leave those and whatever behind to heal and grow, it'll be easier to find peace and comfort in being alone. And this doesn't mean isolation, because you don't want to isolate yourself from the outside world and not explore. There will be times where you will meet new people and partners that are meant for you. It may not be forever, but it's a cycle you have to change and learn from. At times there are karmic cycles or other cycles where people are drawn into your life. Knowing what is the cause of being drawn to non-stable individuals into your life is different for everyone. Everybody signs and generational curses are different, so for one to break a generational curse is difficult. It takes a strong individual to break the barrier and change the lifespan of the next generation in the family. This is moving on and this is making big decisions. Being able to stand up and say "I've had enough" with your actions and less words.

Chapter 8

Big Decisions

Making Big Decisions is being available to a new life. There are many different ways to make big decisions and each decision will bring affect to life. It can be attending a new school, building a business, learning how to cook, or even traveling the world. It's opening your mind and expanding to the universe, though not every decision will be set in stone. When making big decisions, be prepared for the consequences that come with the action done. It could be positive; it could be negative depending on what's done.

The different type of Big Decisions:

Relationships:

Big decisions can be relationships, and committing to being married plays a big role in life. Giving up most of your freedom to finally settle down and feel the love between not only you but also your partner. Being in a relationship (and marriage) means to both grow together, and educate each on one's strengths and knowledge. To be loyal, supportive and sexual (if that's your choice), commitment is huge and it takes both to have a serious conversation to go forward with the relationship. Not every relationship will be loyal between the two, as you may have spent a lot of time with your partner. Don't build high expectations and don't expect every partner who you are in a relationship with to last. Some may cheat, some may become uninterested and unhappy, some may be abusive, and some may let others determine how they feel and control the relationship between you and them. Which is your responsibility to make a move despite the circumstances and love towards your relationship. Do not stay and expect sympathy from others when you are choosing to be in a relationship with no romance and someone who is abusive. Do not complain about your partner and spread misinformation while you are still committed to your partner. Do not tell your business about you or between your partners to anyone else. This means your mother, father, friends (and best friends) no one should know because a relationship should be private but not secretive. A relationship is meant for peace and happiness, this doesn't mean relying on your partner for happiness and comfort. But to enjoy their presence and peace with being around them. If you are not stable in any kind of way, do not enter a relationship. Or use anyone else for rebound purposes because of your last relationship or anything else. Before committing to a relationship, think logically and not with your feelings and heart. Because only thinking with your feelings and heart will only lead you the wrong way. You can make a big decision and commit, but remember not everyone is loyal and deserves your love. Protect your heart and set boundaries to live by. Boundaries should never be ignored or dropped for one person, yet alone any person.

Family:

We all have family relatives we know and may not know. We may even build our own families and feel as one. Which is what this is all about, building a family. Commitment is also being focused on having children and being more than just one person. It's having more than just one vessel of yourself and carrying a child around for 9 months, then giving birth. Similar to relationships because it's also building Relationships. This is taking things more seriously and allowing your partner to impregnate you. Children are expensive so making decisions like getting pregnant and building a stronger bond with your partner should be discussed.

Finance:

Decisions can be made with financial independence or financial responsibility. To buy a property, house, and car is a financial choice of a decision. When making an investment you should be prepared financially for the outcomes and funds it comes down to paying. Yes, make an investment and invest but always be prepared for that investment and not live a life of lies to fulfill others. "Fake it till you make it" as constantly said, but faking financial and a personal interest investment is not worth living a life paying back in debt and taxes you'll owe in the end. So be careful when making big decisions and don't bankrupt your bank account either.

Education:

Getting into a new class or college is not easy. Redoing a course and relearning research on a subject or work environment takes a lot of dedication and effort. Education is important and don't let anyone tell you otherwise. You may not like school or class or a new major but it does pay off in situations where you will need it. To become a teacher, nurse, doctor, electrician and even a pilot requires a lot of study. Many Jobs require a lot of studying and degrees to progress.

So, get the right education needed and required for a Job or Career you want to accomplish.

Career:

Entering a new career is like relearning skills and going back to school. Because you are starting new and different. Some careers require a degree and certification of completion before hiring.

So, it's best to make sure you have everything needed before applying for certain jobs or positions in life. Not everything is perfect and quality work, so it's important to do research on a career or position before walking in a certain path. Some careers are no turning back and others are easy to switch from. Be sure of what career challenges and opportunities you are taking. You may have to move for a Job or learn different languages and cultures skills and hobbies to continue that certain career. Be ready to show who you are and what you are capable of doing to improve yourself and the environment around you.

Maturity:

Growing up is what everyone does physically, but some may not grow mentally and emotionally. And having a maturity level mindset sure will take you to great places instead of the children's spot. There are cases where you can be up of age but still act like a child and never grow mentally. This is called "Arrested Psychology Development", caused by trauma leaving a marking mood after traumatic events. "Arrested Psychology Development" or (APD), impairs the ability to identify and develop full emotions maturity. Leaving the effects of not understanding emotions and others, relationships and more. Though some individuals may not be affected by Arrested Psychology Development (APD). But most individuals are in this is the need for therapy. Making a decision is to commit and understand what's around you. And without fixing inner problems there is no maturing and comprehension to issues that may need to be solved. So, take lessons and experiences to mature from and be around those who are intelligent enough to teach.

Chapter 9

Opening New Doors

Now closing the old doors and leaving the toxins behind. New opportunities are awaiting and rewards to come. Now that we have moved on from old habits and closed old doors, we have become better and healthier from the past. This is where things start to unravel for us and we see better things that our eyes can lay on. New doors for us can be anything, it's anything that's different but also positive in a certain way. And New doors for us can also be different but negative in a certain way. For example, being given an opportunity for a new job or gaining well in peace. As well as establishing relationships can all be beneficial. There are a lot of experiences we will all experience. But the way each experience may go will be different towards each person. So do not expect for one person's experience to be the same as another or yours. Be yourself and what's for you will come to you.

Chapter 10

Still Healing

We will never stop healing for as long as we live. And as we die, we will still be forever healing in the afterlife. There is no such thing as "done healing" because as we heal and grow stronger each and every day. We will always experience interactions that will impact us while we are healing. Interactions can consciously affect us with our own notice and interactions can unconsciously affect us without noticing. Small or big interactions we experience will never be forgotten. Our brains still store memories of things that happened in our life. Likely at times it's difficult to retrieve and find those memories. There is more than one way to find a memory, so do not think healing is all about forgetting. Healing is all about forgiveness, peace, acceptance, understanding, unity and love. It doesn't matter how many people you remove in your life. If your heart is not pure and you are not respectful, then you are the problem. There may have been people out in the world who have hurt you but you also have hurt them in some kind of way. This doesn't justify their actions and your actions but knowledge the behavior between you and them. If no peace is brought to the situation you leave without speaking a word. Healing isn't just about speaking about issues or "healing" from a relationship. It's about understanding and moving forward with forgiveness. You can heal from many things but it takes progress. You can heal from self-harm or trauma or even events that are so deep and painful it leaves a mark on your character. It's only up to you if you want to continue healing and feel the pain needed to be lifted from darkness. It's only you who can help yourself, and others who can support you. But the only support and love those matters is yours, because there is only one of you and only you know yourself more than anybody else, whether you know it or not.

To begin healing if you haven't, it's best to remove the triggers that you are healing from. Example, if you are healing from a traumatic event, any relationship, or other. You want to remove what's causing you to be triggered or to relapse again. Know Relapse isn't failure, but a mistake to learn from. It's not the end of the world if you relapse from any healing you are working on. But it's important to learn from that mistake and reset your mindset to something positive. Be more cautious of your thoughts and actions. If you wake up and have a taste for something sweet. Would you eat it right then? If the answer is yes, then you aren't thinking cautiously. Before you would want something sweet you should ask yourself if you had washed up, made your bed, drank water, ate breakfast, and the normal. A cautious person would simply ask these questions before taking action. It's important that everyone be cautious and aware of what they are doing and when. Though many are never cautious and aware, be careful and mindful of your surroundings and even yourself. Sometimes it is good to watch videos of what someone is going through the same as you. This is because finding a similar situation can help you through and encourage your healing process. Not only this but tell yourself how you feel and explain to yourself why you feel a certain way, you can also tell a trusted therapist if needed. Keep track of your days and emotions of how you feel. Start a check in, to record how your day went and what you did on that day. Trust in yourself and pray to God (if you are religious). Surround yourself with others and not isolate yourself. It's okay to feel uncomfortable and upset about your pain, you are healing. Do not go back to what hurt you and made you suffer just because you are lonely and attached. This is part of the process, and re-identifying yourself to know who you truly are. Listen to music that gives you comfort but not despair in your thoughts. This means to not drown yourself in your thoughts but to feel comfort instead. Everything will be alright.

Chapter 11

Awaking Of the Mindset

Awake your mind and let yourself feel free. Do not keep your mind in a cage and be closed minded. You should be open minded and be able to consider new ideas to enjoy. Because the more you experience new ideas, you will be able to know what you are interested in. You will see new opportunities coming your way, but you should always also have discipline in the way you are opening your mind. To have discipline in awaking your mind means to learn, let go, and know what you have to work on. The way to awaken your mind is to know your problems. You cannot discipline yourself without the knowledge of your problems. The same way as you are healing is the same way of discipline to turn the pain into peace. For your life's sake, everyone and everyday will not bring you peace only because you "open your mind". You will come across those who are not stable at times, and no you do not have to teach them but sometimes it is better to ignore them. Know your worth and do not tolerate disappointment and disrespect.

Keep in mind that you do not need to respond to everything. It is best to notice things and see what you do not like but never to always respond to it. The more you observe, the more you will see. The less you talk, the more you will notice and feel. Let's say you are out or a student still in school, have you ever noticed how other students and or people speak so much and tell their business out loud? You ever feel the differences when you're constantly opening your mouth and telling others your business. Or sometimes when you speak so much you stop paying attention to your surroundings and become less aware of danger if it comes around. Or maybe you notice there are those who do not speak so much or even at all. It is good and bad to communicate, though the good is to communicate with those you know and trust. The bad is to communicate with those who don't listen and don't converse back. You have to notice the difference between who listens and who doesn't listen. For example, you have those who will listen to you and make you feel comfortable with what you are saying. And speak when needed to respond and entertain the conversation. You may also notice their body language and see how they're relaxed and not very tense. You may even have the feeling that they are listening too, and your gut feeling telling you that everything is alright. And then you have those who just listen to be nosy and speak to influence the bad. They are usually always obsessed with your life and angry when they don't know anything about what's going on in your life and or not the first to know. Their body language will always seem to be tense or sometimes their body language can still appear calm and relaxed. They can still be respectful and friendly, but secretly are not your friend, you have to really observe and see what they are. You have some who overly compliment you, and not many seem to notice these kinds of people because they think it's just being "nice" and "supportive" from their friend. This is not true, the type of friends will be explained shortly in another chapter, but remember awakening your mind means to see, observe, and reconnect with your inner self.

Chapter 12

Relaxation

After the hard times and challenges you've been through, it's time to rest. It's time to take a mental break and relax your mind. Rather its personal, work, school, & even more. Just take some time to yourself and relax your mind. Let yourself feel relaxed and maybe even take a reflection on everything that happened. Not to feel sorrow but to process everything and understand. See, our minds need a break too and not every break has to be a reflection. When taking a mind break, turn off music, turn off socials and get off the phone, and sometimes you need to get off a book. Not saying to get off of this book, but when it's time to relax the mind just sit in silence the best you can and it doesn't always have to be at home. You can sit outside and feel and listen to nature. Whatever makes you comfortable, let yourself be comfortable. There are multiple ways to give your mind time to relax. You can lay down, take a breathing break, write about your day, take a walk and more. It's about giving your mind the attention it needs instead of feeding it with unhealthy things. An unhealthy mind can lead to depression and a depression mindset can ultimately lead to death.

So, let's give ourselves the time and resources to stay healthy in the head and remove things that are unhealthy for the mental.

Chapter 13

The Type of Friends

There are supportive friends and there are non-supportive friends, and in this chapter, we will be going over the type of friendships to avoid and relationships as they stand for both.

Jealousy:

Starting off with a common type of friendship will be the jealousy friend. This stands for all things and relationships. The jealous type of friends are usually always trying to knock you down, they tend to give slick comments all the time to try and damage your character. They feel as though you two are always in competition and they want to be the source of attention and attraction. Their facial expressions could also show the opposite of what they are saying and their tone of voice could tell you a lot about their character. Jealous people tend to outdo themselves to seem better and always try to sabotage you or others to be the spotlight. You do not want to be friends with these people but instead keep your distance and business to yourself. Usually these are the kinds that don't like hearing any good from those they are jealous about. So, keep it in silence and remove yourself from a jealousy environment.

Obsession:

The friends who are obsessed are the ones you want to watch out for. They are not only obsessed but later they go into a Stalking stage and gradually get worse. Similar to Jealousy, they go through stages and become dangerous to others. And those stages are usually warnings to others, rather cautiously or not. They usually give signs of overly emotional, aggressive, and sometimes violent behavior. This includes always wanting to know where that person is at all times. Thinking about that person most of the time and trying to reduce their contact with anyone else but them. These are signs of an obsessed friend. Everyone's signs are different so keep a look for those who are too needy. And remember you are not in a relationship with any of your friends, so don't treat your friends as your boyfriend or girlfriend. That's only for relationships and yes, there is a difference between helping a friend and a friend being too needy. When you are helping a friend, you are helping them get back on their feet and to be able to do things back on their own. It's supporting your friends and making sure they are on the right track. Then those who are too needy tend to need "help" for everything. And start to rely more upon a person and expect everything to be done by them. Don't let anybody rely on you and don't rely on anyone yourself. Remove those obsessive friends.

Messy and gossip:

Friends who are messy are always in drama and if you didn't know. They are usually the ones who start drama, it may be amusing to hear about somebody's else's life and what's going on. But it's none of your business, and unfortunately many fails to understand that. Would you like your business being spread out and everyone knowing what's going on in your life? No, you wouldn't and friends who do that don't even have their own life. People who have things to do don't worry about anyone else's life. Because they don't care and are too involved on their own. And if you are surrounded by people and friends who are involved in modern tea (drama). You need to leave, because you will not get anywhere in life by involving yourself into others' lives and dealing with those who like to gossip. Keep your business and life private so you can grow and work towards your goals. Friends who like to gossip will always have opinions and will be the one to spread your business faster than anything and anyone.

Secretly copying you:

Being friends sometimes we don't notice that they secretly copy us. And friends who secretly copy you may stem from insecurity and don't know their identity. This is not to say "help them find their identity" but to remove yourself from somebody who doesn't know their identity and is very insecure. Because insecure people push their insecurities onto others and want to make them feel bad as well. This is toxic and is very overlooked in friendships. They may copy off your clothes, the way you speak, makeup, how you present yourself and more. And if that friend is really smart, they will try and copy your personality and switch things around so that you can't say they "copy" you. They're sneaky and just like manipulators, they'll turn things around and make little changes so you won't notice. And for friends who are petty and want you to know their coping, will send hints for you to catch on. This is to be disrespectful because they want to shove it in your face.

So, if you have friends who copy off of you, remove them and find better ones.

Feeling uncomfortable around them:

Would you like to stay friends with someone who makes you feel uncomfortable? Well, I suppose no. Because when you become friends with someone it is okay to be a little shy around them and a little uncomfortable. You are getting to know that person and figure out what you both have in common. But after a while that feeling of shyness and awkwardness goes away. Where now you two are comfortable around each other as friends. But sometimes we may have come across people where we felt uncomfortable no matter what. And we could have known that person for a long time or quite some weeks or months. But even if you know that person for a few years or less, you shouldn't feel so uncomfortable around them. If you do feel uncomfortable around someone, you can speak to them about it or leave the friendship. You don't have to stay in a friendship where you feel uncomfortable. Put yourself first and stand your ground.

They lie:

You don't want to be friends with a person who lies a lot. Because they will lie about anything. It could be a simple question or a simple conversation. For example, you could ask what that friend ate and they'll lie and say "nothing". Knowing they ate before or you could ask if they have a charger and they'll say "no" knowing they have a charger and go charge their phone after lying in your face. That's petty and rude behavior. These kinds of friends do it on purpose to be rude in the friendship, they don't respect you. There would be no reason to lie unless it's a situation where it's life or death. People who lie a lot are also manipulators, and manipulation is used in a lot of tactics and lying is one of them. There would be no reason to lie about such a simple thing or anything in general. Imagine being in a situation where it's important and your friend lies about something serious. How would you feel? Because your friend who lied obviously didn't care and definitely didn't care since they thought about the lie and said it straight to your face. You have to look at certain things on a certain level and ask yourself. Should I be friends with this person? Or in general of what you're doing. Ask yourself, "Is this worth it?" Because if your answer is No to both questions. Then what are you doing and why are you friends with that person? Friends should respect each other and have no reason to lie.

Bad influence:

A negative attitude will get you nowhere. And being with a friend who is negative will lead you in the wrong direction. Being negative is the same as a bad influence, because negativity influences our attitude and actions. And in an environment where its always negativity comes from bad influence. Nothing good comes out of a bad influence and don't get comfortable with those who are a bad influence. Because sooner you will be easily influenced and manipulated to do things that will not benefit you. Sometimes those who are a bad influence come from bad environments and people who didn't take care of them when they were younger. Though it's up to you if you want to stay knowing that they are a bad influence and negative towards others. A person cannot control how they were raised when younger but a person can control their actions and behavior. And usually, an influence knows what they are doing but they just don't care. A person who is negative, also knows that they are negative but again they just don't care. And it's not up to you to make them care but instead to remove yourself because they don't care. And a person who doesn't care what they are doing and what influence they have on others, doesn't care about themselves and those around them.

Chapter 14

Isolation

Isolation is powerful and can help us in situations where we have to realize what's around us and about ourselves. Isolation can be positive and negative depending on how you are isolating yourself. Do not isolate yourself from everyone and everything, but do it to your extended point. Meaning, do it as long as you feel you need to. Sometimes when reality is harsh, we have no choice but to isolate ourselves and work on what has to be changed. This can lead to cutting off people who we thought would stay in our lives, moving away, not doing your dream career and more. This is usually because something better is for us and to attend and attract what's better for us we have to make changes ourselves and prepare ourselves for the best. But don't worry about the future but instead work on yourself in your present. Because what you do in the present is your future, how you are acting, thinking and your environment all contribute to your future. Because we don't know what's for us in the future, but how we are acting in our present will give us our future. So be careful with what you are doing and how you are doing something.

How do we isolate ourselves? And is isolating ourselves worth it? Isolating ourselves can help us understand more about our identity and who we are. It shows us our flaws and imperfections to take a deeper look at and to figure out what we have to change. Each of us have our own way of isolation and with what works best for us.

So, know what best isolation technique works for you. When isolating yourself, understand some people will leave and be cut off. And understand that this does not mean to just disappear without telling others you at least want to take a break to be with yourself. Unless you want to disappear without telling anyone that is your choice. You can isolate yourself as long as you want but this is to better yourself and understand more about yourself. This is not to be negative and neglect your mental health of what's important. But when you isolate yourself, understand once you start to go back out, meet people and explore places. Your perspective will be different and you will start to realize many things. You will be more comfortable with being alone and not worrying about nobody else. You will start to want and have more peace. People will still talk about you regardless or wonder about you but that is none of your business. Because if there is no peace with what you are doing, why are you doing it? Or if you are talking to someone where you two always argue and there is no peace in between. Why are you still talking to them? Once you go into isolation and find peace and love within yourself. It will be harder to let another person bring you down and easier for you to not care and cut them off with no problem. And for those who are Religious, know what you are doing. Do it with God because with God all things are possible.

Chapter 15

Perspectives

   Situations and words of what people say can change our perspective. As our perspectives are changed it's changed forever, never temporary. When our perspectives change, our minds change too and this helps us to grow and become more wise. Sometimes things happen to show us a lesson and other times it's to show us a good time. We will go through things that will hurt us or make us feel some type of way but you have to choose how to handle the situation and keep your composure. This also helps us to know what to look out for in the future, future situations or events. It's okay to feel upset when something, someone you use to look at a certain way now changes. Everyone changes and it's a part of our growth, so do not expect everything or everyone to always stay the same. Love yourself, because the way we see things is important, it shifts us as a whole individual to become someone new. So don't be afraid of change and lesson learning, but instead be grateful and prepared. Being grateful and prepared will help you know what's coming and to not disappoint yourself. People will disappoint you and do unexpected things.

So, see them as they are and nothing else, nothing more or nothing less. Not everyone is going to stay in your life either, or respect you. There are many things you will experience and see in life. Parents sometimes prepare us for the world and some may not. There will be times where you have to teach yourself about your own perspective, intelligence, new skills and more. like it says in chapters, not everyone will be there to save you.

What can change our perspective? There are many things that can change our perspective. It could be relationships, hurtful situations, movies, a conversation and even more. Each of us has something that has changed us in some kind of way. But how we handle that situation in our life matters the most. Because the more we practice with understanding and having control with what we can control. When we get older, we will become more successful because we already know how to handle these situations and emotions. And people will not like you because of that, though this doesn't mean to change who you are. Because you won't be liked regardless by others. You have to accept yourself and forgive yourself before doing the same for anyone else. Because that's how we grow and how our perspective can change. The interest in our old habits and people will not be the same anymore. Our interests would stem to more new habits and our view processes would be more different. This can also help us to mature more, especially for those who haven't yet matured enough to understand certain things. Age doesn't matter when it comes to deep topics, because anyone can experience something deep or a life lesson. It can be hard on us at times too, to have to realize and see certain things that we wish we couldn't have seen or known about. But everything happens for a reason and we as individuals are on this planet called "earth" to learn and gain knowledge.